Anti-Inflammatory Diet Cookbook

Become Healthy and Revitalize Yourself. Easy and Delicious Anti Inflammatory Recipes

Lulu Calimeris

Disclaimer

The content, writing, images, photos, descriptions and information contained in this book are for general guidance and are intended for informational purposes only for the readers. The author has narrated his cooking and research experiences in this book by observing and evaluating relevant facts and figures. The author is not a registered dietitian and nutritional information in this book should only be used as a general guideline. Statements in this book have not been evaluated or approved by any regulatory authority.

The author has tried to provide all the information related to the ingredients, foods, and products, however, when certain ingredients get mixed, they may create some kind of cross-reaction which may cause allergy among some people. There may be products that will not be gluten-free and may contain ingredients that may cause a reaction. These products may include but are limited to, eggs, dairy, wheat, nuts, coconut, flour, soy, cocoa, milk, sugar, and other products. These may cause allergic reactions in some people due to cross-contamination from allergen-causing products. The readers and purchasers of this book understand and consent that there may be ingredients in the foods which may contain certain allergens and the readers and purchasers hereby disclaimer the author of this book from all liabilities related to allergic and cross food reactions.

The information provided in this book must not be taken as an alternative to any advice by a doctor, physician, dietitian or health care specialist. The readers should not use the information given in this book for diagnosing an illness or other health-related problems. Furthermore, the readers also should not discontinue professional medical or healthcare advice because of something they have read in this book. The content and information provided in this book do not create any kind of professional relationship between the reader and the author of this book.

This book in no way provides any warranty, express or implied, towards the content of recipes contained in this book. It is the reader's responsibility to determine the value and quality of any recipe or instructions provided for food preparation and to determine the nutritional value if any, and safety of the preparation instructions. Therefore, the author of this book is not responsible for the outcome of any recipe that a reader may try from this book. The readers of this book may not always have the same results due to variations in ingredients, humidity, altitude, cooking temperatures, errors, omissions, or individual cooking abilities.

The images and photos contained in this book may have been used for representational, informative and information purposes and may not be the exact match of the accompanying recipes. These images and photos provide the author's impression of how a particular recipe might look after it has been cooked, made or completed and the images and photos should only be relied upon for the purpose of reference and not actual finished products, recipes or foods.

By purchasing this book, readers hereby acknowledge that they are going to rely on any information provided in the book 'as-is' and must not use this information to form any final conclusion, whether the information is in the form of description, recipe, or ingredient. Readers agree that they will consult a physician, dietitian or professional healthcare specialist before using and relying on any data, information, or suggestion described in this book. Readers agree to accept all risks of relying upon and using any of the information presented in this book. Readers also agree to hold harmless the author, editor, publisher, affiliates, team, and staff members or anyone associated with this book from and against any damages, lawsuits, costs, claims, expenses including any legal fees, medical fees, or insurance fees resulting from the application of any of the information provided by this book. Any reliance readers make on any information presented in this book is at their sole discretion and risk. The author of this book hereby disclaims any liability in connection with the use of any information presented in this book.

Table of Contents

Anti-inflammatory Dinner Recipes

Cranberry And Orange Balls

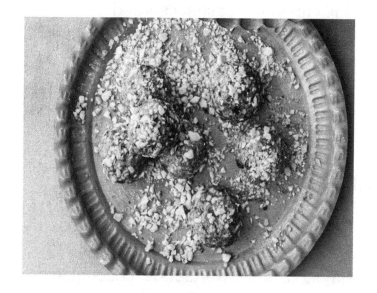

Prep Time: 50 minutes
Cook Time: 0 minute
Servings: 20 people

Ingredients

- 12 medjool dates pitted
- 2 teaspoons of the honey
- 2 teaspoons of the finely grated orange rind
- Half cup of the cashew spread
- Half cup of the linseed, sunflower seeds and almonds
- 4 tablespoons of the shredded coconut
- 4 tablespoons of the cranberries
- ¾ cup of the pistachio kernels

Directions

- Take a food processor and add the dates, orange rind, cashew spread, Linseeds, almonds, sunflower seeds, coconut flakes, cranberries and 4 tablespoons of the pistachios. Let them pulse until they are well combined and coarse mixture is formed
- Then finely chop the remaining pistachios and then place them in the separate bowl
- Now roll the pulsed mixture in ball form and then roll on them in the pistachios mixture to lightly coat them
- Then place these balls in the plate
- Let them refrigerate for about 20 minutes
- Serve them and enjoy

Green Leaf Salad With Strawberry Balsamic Vinaigrette

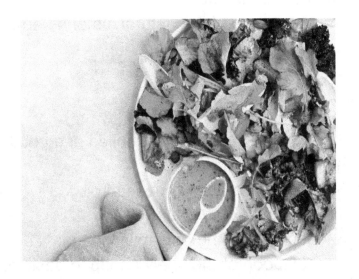

Prep Time: 15 minutes
Cook Time: 0 minute
Servings: 4 people

Ingredients

- 1 yellow witlof leaves separated
- 1 bunch of the rocket trimmed
- 3 stalks of the red kale leaves finely chopped
- 125 grams of the strawberries, hulled and then cut them in halved
- 4 tablespoons of the natural almond kernels toasted

Strawberry Balsamic Vinaigrette

- 1 cup of the strawberries, hulled and cut them half sized
- 3 teaspoons of the grapeseed oil
- 1 tablespoon of the honey
- 3 teaspoons of the balsamic vinegar
- 1 tablespoon of the finely chopped basil leaves

Directions

- First of all make the strawberry balsamic vinaigrette. Place the strawberries, oil, honey, and vinegar in the bowl, pulse them until they are smooth
- Then season them with some salt and pepper. Then stir them in the basil leaves
- Then place the witlof, rocket, kale, strawberries and almonds on a serving plate
- Drizzle them with some dressing

- Then serve them and enjoy

Festive Fruit Salad

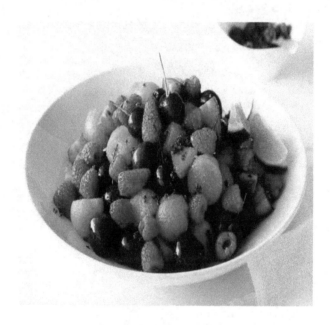

Prep Time: 15 minutes
Cook Time: 0 minute
Servings: 4 people

Ingredients

- 400 grams of the cherries
- 250 grams of the strawberries cut then in half sized
- 125 grans of the strawberries
- 125 grams of the raspberries
- 2 tablespoons of the finely chopped mint leaves
- 2 tablespoons of the caster sugar
- ¼ of the watermelon
- 2 teaspoons of the lemon juice

Directions

- Take a large bowl add the strawberries, raspberries and cherries. Then take a melon baller and cut the watermelon in the cube shape
- Then add then in the bowl
- Then combine the mint leaves and sugar in the small bowl
- Use the end of the rolling pin to crush the mint and sugar
- Then sprinkle only half of the mint sugar over the fruits
- And squeeze them lemon juice over the fruits
- Then toss them to combine let them set aside for about 10 minutes until the syrup develops

- Then serve them by sprinkling the mint sugar over them
- Then serve them and enjoy

Salmon And Fennel Salad

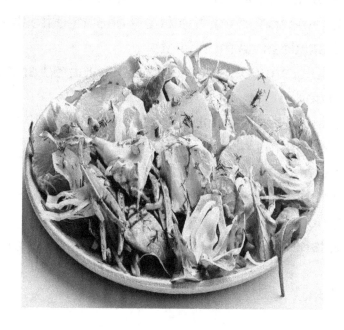

Prep Time: 1 hour and 20 minutes
Cook Time: 10 minutes
Servings: 6 people

Ingredients

- 4 oranges
- 1 tablespoon of the finely grated lemon rind
- 2 tablespoons of the Dijon mustard
- 2 tablespoons of the finely chopped fresh dill
- 3 skinless salmon fillets
- 250 grams of the snow peas trimmed and thinly sliced
- 2 baby fennel bulbs, trimmed and thinly sliced
- 120 grams of the baby spinach
- Some rocket leaves for salad
- 1 tablespoon of the white wine balsamic vinegar
- 2 tablespoons of the finely chopped pistachios

Directions

- Take a bowl and finely grated the lemon rind, orange rind, mustard, half of the orange juice, and 1 tablespoon of the dill, in a shallow dish
- Then add the salmon in then let them coat
- Then let them cover and place them in the refrigerator for about 1 hour to marinate
- Preheat the chargrill on medium heat
- Then drain the marinade from the salmon and spray them with so keep olive oil
- Then cook the salmon for about 3 minutes by flipping from each side

- Then set them aside and let them cool
- Then coarsely flake the salmon
- Then put the snow peas in the heat proof bowl, let them cover with the boiling water and set then aside
- Then refresh them by using the cold water and then set them aside
- Take a large bowl add the snow peas, fennel, salad leaves, and orange slices. Whisk the vinegar, extra mustard, remaining orange juice, and try remaining dill in the bowl. Then add half of the salad dressing to the bowl
- Then toss them to coat well and combine
- Then pile the salad on the serving plate, then top them with the salmon, drizzle them with the remaining salad dressing and then sprinkle them with the chopped pistachios
- Serve them and enjoy

Turkey Couscous Pilaf

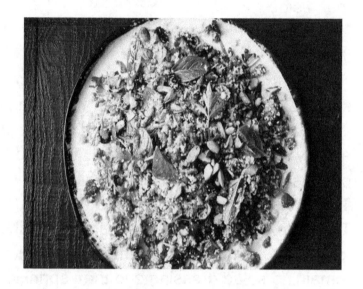

Prep Time: 20 minutes
Cook Time: 20 minutes
Servings: 4 people

Ingredients

- 2 teaspoons of the extra virgin olive oil
- 1 small sized red onion finely chopped
- 2 minced garlic cloves
- 2 teaspoons of the ground cumin powder
- 2 teaspoons of the ground coriander powder
- 1 tablespoon of the grated ginger
- Half teaspoon of the ground cinnamon powder
- ¼ teaspoon of the ground chilli powder/ flakes
- 500 grams of the minced turkey
- 1 cup of the couscous
- Half cup of the dried cranberries
- 1 tablespoon of the lemon rind
- 1 teaspoon of the lemon juice
- 1 cup of the boiling water
- 1 cup of the fresh mint leaves
- 1 cup of the fresh coriander leaves
- 2 tablespoons of the chopped pistachios toasted
- Some extra virgin olive oil

Directions

- Take a nonstick pan add some olive oil let them heat up then add the onions and garlic stir then continuously until they are tendered or turned into golden brown

- Then add the ground cinnamon powder, cumin powder, ground cinnamon powder and chilli powder
- Let them cook while continuously stirring for about 1 minute
- Then increase the heat to high flame and then add the turkey in them
- Let them cook by using wooden spoon and continuously breaking until they are tendered or turned into golden brown
- Take a heatproof bowl and add couscous, cranberries, lemon rind, juice and water. Then let then cover with a plastic wrap
- Let them set aside form about 5 minutes until they are absorbed
- Then fluff them by using a fork
- Then finely chop half of the the mint leaves and coriander. Then add the turkey mixture and the mint and coriander to the couscous
- Stir them to combine, then sprinkle them with chopped pistachios and then drizzle them with the extra virgin olive oil
- Then serve them and enjoy

Roasted Pumpkin Salad With Cranberries And Pistachios

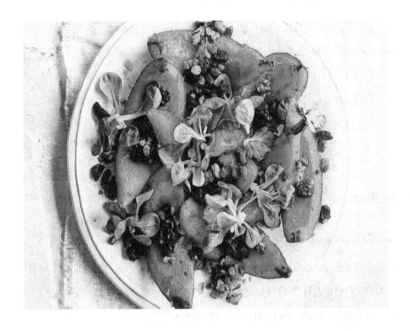

Prep Time: 10 minutes
Cook Time: 40 minutes
Servings: 8 people

Ingredients

- 1 small sized pumpkin let them cut in wedges
- 80 ml of the filtered water
- 2 tablespoons of the maple syrup
- 1 teaspoon of the smoked paprika
- 1 minced garlic clove
- 3 tablespoons of the extra virgin olive
- 80 grams of the dried cranberries
- 50 grams of the chopped pistachios
- 50 grams of the chopped salad leaves
- Some freshly chopped coriander leaves
- 1 tablespoon of the lemon juice

Directions

- Preheat an oven at 350 degrees F
- Take a baking tray lined with the parchment paper and grease then with some olive oil
- Place the pumpkin in the tray
- Season them lightly with some salt and black pepper
- Take a hug add water, maple syrup, paprika powder, garlic, and extra virgin olive oil
- Sprinkle some salt and black pepper in them
- Stir them to combine and then drizzle them on the pumpkin
- Let them roast for about 30 minutes until they are tendered

- Then add the pistachios and cranberries in the pan and let them roast for about 5 minutes more
- Then transfer them to the serving plate and top with the salad leaves and coriander
- Then combine the rest of the oil and lemon juice then drizzle over the salad
- Serve them and enjoy

Chia, Quinoa And Buckwheat Bread

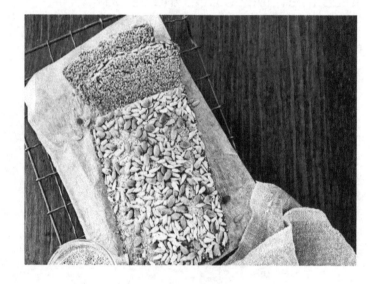

Prep Time: 2 hours 15 minutes
Cook Time:1 hour 20 minutes
Servings: 12 people

Ingredients

- 1 cup of the Brazil nuts
- 3 tablespoons of the chia seeds
- 2 cups of the white quinoa
- 1 cup of the sunflower seeds
- Half cup of the almond meal
- Some pinch of salt
- 2 tablespoons of the coconut oil
- 2 tablespoons of the honey
- 1 ½ cups of the water
- 1 tablespoon of the pepitas
- 1 tablespoon of the sunflower seeds

Directions

- Take a food processor and add the Brazil nuts and buckwheat let them process until they are coarsely chopped
- Then transfer them to the large bowl and add chia seeds, quinoa, sunflower seeds, almond meal, coconut oil, honey and water
- Stir them until they are well combined together
- Then set them aside for 1 hour and 30 minutes
- Let them stir halfway through
- Preheat an oven at 350 degrees F
- Take 9 cm deep loaf pan and greased them with some olive oil

- Then line the baking pan with the parchment paper
- Let them extend above the edges of the pan
- Spoon the buckwheat mixture in the pan then let them press the mixture by using the back of the spoon
- Add the rest of the buckwheat mixture and then sprinkle on them pepitas and sunflower seeds pressing them to secure
- Let them bake for about 1 hour then reduce the oven temperature and again bake them for about 20 minutes
- Then remove them and let them cool down for 10 minutes
- Then lift the bread up and serve them
- Enjoy

Roasted Vegetables And Buckwheat Salad

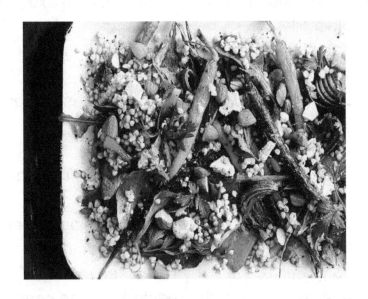

Prep Time: 10 minutes
Cook Time: 25 minutes
Servings: 4 people

Ingredients

- 2 bunches of the baby rainbow carrot, let them trimmed and scrubbed
- 2 red capsicum coarsely chopped
- 1 red onion cut them in wedges
- 2 tablespoons of the Cobram Estate extra virgin olive oil
- 4 tablespoons of the orange juice
- 1 teaspoon of the cumin seeds
- 2 teaspoons of the finely grated fresh ginger
- 1 minced garlic clove
- 2 tablespoons of the honey
- 200 grams of the raw buckwheat, rinsed and dried
- 1 cup of the freshly chopped parsley leaves
- 100 grams of the feta cheese crumbled
- 40 grams of the baby rocket leaves
- 4 tablespoons of the roasted almond coarsely chopped

Directions

- Preheat an oven at 450 degrees F
- Take a baking tray lined with parchment paper and spray with some olive oil
- Scatter the veggies over the baking tray, then drizzle some of the olive oil
- Season them with salt and pepper to taste

- Then let then roast for about 15 minutes
- Then take a bowl add the orange juice, cumin seeds, ginger, garlic, and some honey. Stir them to combine well
- Then drizzle them over the veggies
- Then let then roast turning halfway through and let them roast for about 20 minutes more until they are tendered
- Take a nonstick pan add some oil and then add the buckwheat in them let them cook for about 2 minutes while continuously stirring until they are tendered
- Then allow them to cool down and then bring a saucepan of water to boil and then let them heat up and then add the buckwheat to the pan, let them simmer for about 5 minutes until they are tendered
- Let them drain and refresh under the cold running water
- Then spread them on the baking tray lined with the parchment paper
- Take a bowl add the remaining honey, oil and vinegar. Stir them to combine well then season them with some salt and black pepper to taste
- Then add the buckwheat, crumbled feta cheese, herbs, roasted veggies, and rocket
- Toss them to combine, then divide them in plates, then top them with the almonds
- Then serve them and enjoy

Broccoli With Anchovy Almonds

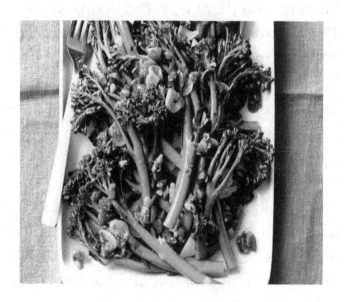

Prep Time: 5 minutes
Cook Time: 5 minutes
Servings: 6 people

Ingredients

- 1 tablespoon of the extra virgin olive oil
- 2 clove of garlic thinly sliced
- 2 tablespoons of the finely grated lemon rind
- 1 long sized red chilli deseeded and finely chopped
- 4 anchovies in oil chopped
- 4 tablespoons of the coarsely chopped almonds
- 2 tablespoons of the lemon juice
- 2 bunches of the broccolini trimmed

Directions

- Take a nonstick pan add the oil then add the garlic, lemon rind, chilli, and drained anchovies
- Let them cook for about 1 minute while continuously stirring
- Then remove them from the heat and stir in them lemon juice
- Take a steamer basket and set over them the simmering water
- Let them cover and cook them for about 2-3 minutes each until they are tendered or crispy
- Then transfer them to the serving plate
- The top them with the almond mixture
- Serve them and enjoy

Rocket, Avocado And Walnut Salad

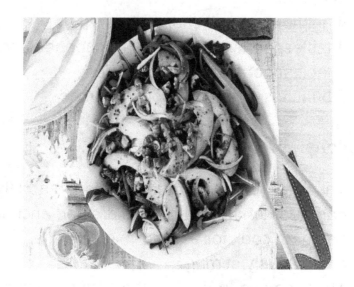

Prep Time: 10 minutes
Cook Time: 5 minutes
Servings: 4 people

Ingredients

- 3 tablespoons of the extra virgin olive oil
- 2 tablespoons of the lemon juice
- 1 teaspoon of the whole grain mustard
- 100 grams of the baby rocket leaves
- Half red onion finely chopped
- 1 avocado peeled and cut them in slices
- Some roasted walnuts for sprinkling

Directions

- Preheat an oven at 459 degrees F
- Take a nonstick pan and spread the walnuts over then let them roast for about 5 minutes by flipping from both sides
- Let them cool down and then coarsely chop them
- Take a small sized screwtop, add the lemon juice, oil and mustard in them
- Season them with salt and pepper. Then shake then to combine
- Take a serving dish and combine the rocket and onions, drizzle them with some dressing and then toss them to combine
- Then top them with the avocado
- And then drizzle them with the remaining dressing
- Scatter over then the roasted walnuts

- Then serve them and enjoy

Mediterranean Oatmeal

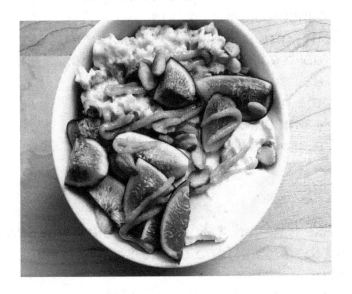

Prep Time: 10 minutes
Cook Time: 5 minutes
Servings: 2 people

Ingredients

- 1 cup of oats (you can choose any of your choice I have chosen old fashioned oats)
- 6 medium sized figs cut into quarters
- 7 ounces of plain yogurt
- Some ground cinnamon powder to taste
- 3 tablespoons of shelled pistachios
- 2 tablespoons of tahini
- Some honey to taste
- 1 teaspoon of Lemon juice
- ⅓ teaspoon of all spices

Directions

- Take a nonstick skillet add water then add oats let them cook for 5 minutes while continuously stirring
- Then cut the figs into quarters
- Take a blender and add the sauce ingredients and blend until smooth
- When the pats will be cooked then add the half of the yogurt and then add the cinnamon powder
- Then transfer the oats to bowl top with the rest of the yogurt, figs and pistachios. Drizzle some tahini sauce and honey
- Serve them and enjoy

Mediterranean Chickpea Salad

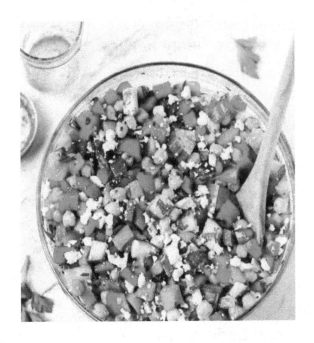

Prep Time: 10 minutes
Cook Time: 15 minutes
Servings: 8 people

Ingredients

Salad

- 1 red onion finely chopped
- 2 cans of chickpeas water drained and rinsed
- 2 cups of fresh leafy parsley
- 1 red bell pepper finely chopped
- 1 small orange and yellow bell peppers finely chopped
- 1 green bell pepper finely chopped
- ½ cucumber peeled and finely chopped
- 4 ounces of the crumbled feta

Dressing

- 2 teaspoons of extra virgin olive oil
- 2 teaspoons of red wine vinegar
- 2 minced garlic cloves
- 2 teaspoons of dried oregano
- Some kosher salt to taste
- Some ground black pepper to taste

Directions

- Take a bowl full of water add the chopped onions let them soak until you prepare the rest of the ingredients it will remove the hasher bite from the onions)

- Now take another bowl add the bell peppers, chickpeas, parsley, cucumbers, and feta
- Now take a small bowl add the dressing ingredients stir them to combine
- Then pour them on the ingredients and add then add the onions
- Toss them to combine well
- Let them bake for about 15 minutes in the oven at 450 degrees F
- Then remove them and serve
- Enjoy

Lentil Salad With Cucumbers

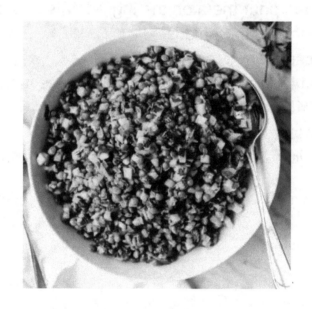

Prep Time: 10 minutes
Cook Time: 20 minutes
Serving: 6 people

Ingredients

- 1 cup of lentils
- 4 cups of the water
- 2 bay leaf
- 1 piece approximately of 3-4 inches kombu
- 1 cucumber in diced form
- 1 small red onion in diced form
- 1 cup of medjool dates in diced form
- ½ cup of finely chopped parsley
- 2 teaspoons of lemon juice

Directions

- Take a bowl add lentils wash then and drain them
- Then take a nonstick skillet add water and then add the water drained lentils, bay leaves, Jonny let them cook on medium flame for about 12 minutes
- Then drain the lentils and let them set aside
- Then take a bowl add the lentils, cucumbers, red onions, dates and parsley
- Them drizzle the lemon juice and toss them to combine
- Then serve them and enjoy

Roasted Beetroots Hummus With Basil Pesto

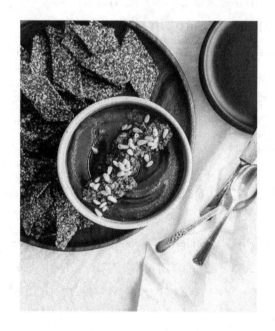

Prep Time: 20 minutes
Cook Time: 60 minutes
Servings: 5 people

Ingredients

- 2 large beetroots
- 2 cups of the cooked chickpeas
- 4 tablespoons of extra virgin olive oil
- 5 tablespoons of tahini sauce
- 5 tablespoons of lemon juice
- 2 minced garlic cloves
- Some salt to taste
- Some ground black pepper to taste
- Some basil pesto as per taste
- ¼ cup of fresh basil leaves
- 2 tablespoons of extra virgin olive oil
- 3 tablespoons of the pine nuts
- 1 minced garlic clove
- Some salt and black pepper to taste

Directions

- Preheat an oven at 450 degrees F
- Take the beetroots, cut their ends and peel them. Then wrap them in the foil and let them bake in the preheated oven
- Bake them for about 1 hour after one hour remove them from the oven and then cut them in slices
- Take a food processor and process them until smooth
- Then transfer then in a bowl

- Then wash the food processor and add the basil pesto ingredients and process them until they are mixed
- Then add the basil pesto on the beetroot hummus and top them with the extra virgin olive oil and pine nuts

Cauliflower Rice Tabbouleh

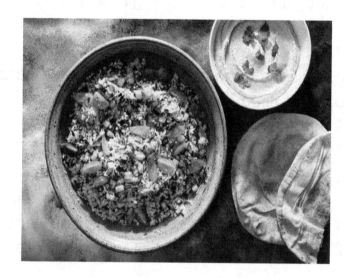

Prep Time: 10 minutes
Cook Time: 15 minutes
Servings: 5 people

Ingredients

- 1 large head of the cauliflower coarsely chopped
- 4 tablespoons of extra virgin olive oil
- Some kosher salt to taste
- 2 cups of the leafy parsley
- 3 scallions (take white and pale green parts only in sliced form)
- 1 minced garlic clove
- 1 tablespoon of lemon zest
- 3 tablespoons of lemon juice
- 1 teaspoon of the crushed red pepper flakes
- 1 small cucumber cut into bite-sized pieces
- 2 cups of the cherry tomatoes cut into half sized

Directions

- Take a food processor and add the coarsely chopped cauliflower. Let them process in the food processor until it turns into rice form
- Then add them in the oven safe bowl and sprinkle some salt and olive oil. Toss them to combine all the ingredients together then microwave them for 3 minutes by covering them bowl with the foil
- Then after 3 minutes remove the foil and spread the cauliflower rice on the rimmed baking sheet and let them cool

- Now clean the food processor and add the parsley, mint, garlic, scallions, lemon juice, lemon zest, salt and olive oil. Let them process until they are chopped or processed finely
- Transfer these ingredients in a bowl and stir in the red pepper flakes
- Then add the cucumbers, cauliflower and tomatoes. Toss then to combine all the ingredients together until well combined
- Then season them with the salt and serve
- Enjoy

Melon Mozzarella Salad

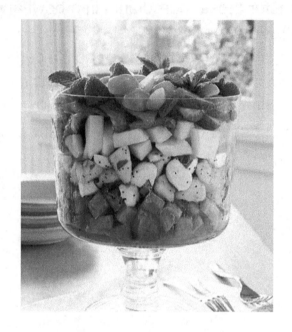

Prep Time: 10 minutes
Cook Time: 20 minted
Servings: 8 people

Ingredients

- 3 cups of freshly peeled peaches in diced form
- 1 tub of fresh mozzarella cheese balls, cut them in half
- 2 tablespoons of the fresh basil leaves
- 3 tablespoons of the lemon poppy seeds dressings
- 5 cups of the watermelon peeled and cut in cube sized
- 4 cups of the honeydew melon
- 3 cups of the freshly sliced strawberries
- 2 cups of the seedless grapes cut in half sized
- Some fresh mint leaves to garnish
- Some fresh raspberries to garnish

Directions

- Take a large sized fruit trifle dish and add the first 3 ingredients with lemon poppy seeds dressings. Toss then until well combined
- Then layer the fruits accordingly
- Let them chill for about 1 hour in the refrigerator
- After that remove them and toss with the rest of the dressings before the serving
- Garnish then with raspberries and mint leaves
- Serve them and enjoy

Sauteed Cabbage

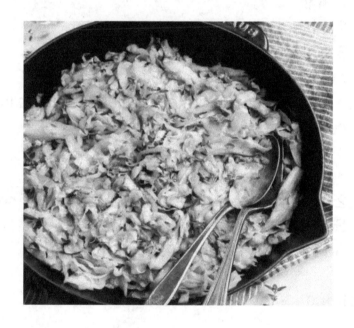

Prep Time: 5 minutes
Cook Time: 10 minutes
Servings: 8 people

Ingredients

- 2 pounds of green cabbage
- 1 tablespoon of the extra virgin olive oil
- 2 tablespoons of the unsalted melted butter
- 2 tablespoons of the kosher salt
- Some freshly ground black pepper
- 1 teaspoon of the apple cider vinegar
- 1 teaspoon of freshly chopped thyme

Directions

- Take a cutting board discard the cabbage core and then thinly slice the cabbage like fine ribbons
- Take a nonstick sauteing pan add the olive oil and butter. Let them heat up.
- Then add the cabbage and sprinkle some salt and black pepper stir them to combine well
- Let them saute for 15 minutes until the cabbage is tendered or softened
- Then remove them from the heat and pour the apple cider vinegar
- Sprinkle some salt and black pepper to taste
- Sprinkle some thyme and serve hot
- Enjoy

Sweet Potato Soup

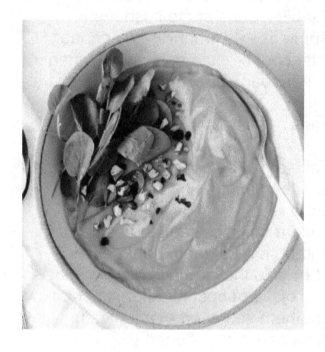

Prep Time: 10 minutes
Cook Time: 30 minutes
Servings: 4 people

Ingredients

- 2 tablespoons of the avocado oil
- 4 small sized carrots sliced
- 1 yellow onion
- 2 pounds of the sweet potato peeled and diced form
- 2 minced garlic cloves
- 1 tablespoon of finely chopped ginger
- ¼ teaspoon of the red chilli flakes
- ¼ teaspoons of paprika powder
- 4 cups of the vegetable broth
- Watercress to garnish
- Some chopped pistachios to garnish
- 1 tablespoon of coconut cream to garnish
- Ground or cracked black pepper to garnish
- Some red pepper flakes to garnish

Directions

- Take a large stock pot and add the olive oil let them heat up
- Then add the carrots and onions let them cook for about 8 minutes while stirring frequently
- Then add the garlic, red pepper flakes, ginger and paprika
- Stir them for 3 minutes until their fragrance comes out
- Then add the vegetable broth and diced sweet potatoes let them boil for 3 minutes on high flame and then let them simmer for 12 minutes
- Then take a high speed blender and add the cooked ingredients in them blend them until

well creamy soup is formed you can add some more vegetables broth if you want
- Pour the soup in a bowl and top with the toppings
- Serve them and enjoy

Beet Soup

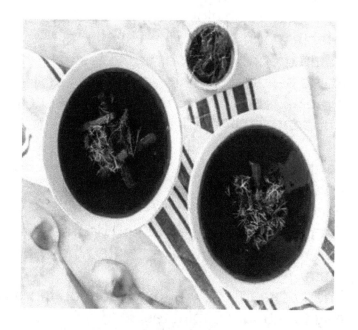

Prep Time: 15 minutes
Cook Time: 45 minutes
Servings: 4 people

Ingredients

- 4 cups of the chicken stock
- 4 whole finely peeled beets
- 1 teaspoon of sugar
- 1 minced garlic clove
- 1 tablespoon of red wine vinegar
- Some ground black pepper to taste
- Some salt to taste
- 4 tablespoons of the mashed boil potatoes
- Chopped basil leaves for garnishing

Directions

- Gather all the ingredients together
- Then preheat an oven at 450 degrees For. Take an aluminum foil and wrap the beets in them
- Then bake them by putting them on the baking tray for about 45 minutes
- After 45 minutes remove them and let them cool for sometime
- Then cut the beet roots in julienne
- Now take a medium pot add the chicken stock and let them boil
- Then add the sliced beets, lemon juice, garlic, sugar, salt and black pepper
- Let them simmer for about 10 minutes
- Then pour the soup in the bowl serve them hot by garnishing it with boiled potatoes and chopped basil leaves
- Enjoy

Salmon Patties

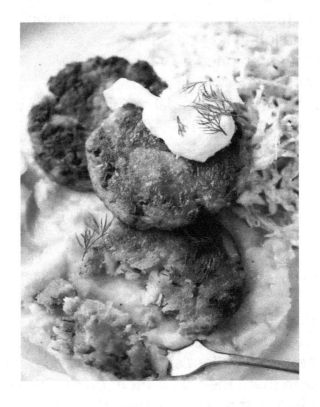

Prep Time: 15 minutes
Cook Time: 20 minutes
Servings: 4 people

Ingredients

- 1 ½ cups of the panko breadcrumbs
- 1 small sized grated onion
- 1 minced garlic clove
- 15 ounces of the cooked pink salmon
- 2 shallots finely sliced
- 2 green onions finely grated
- 2 scallions finely sliced
- ½ cup of the fresh dill roughly chopped
- 2 golden eggs whisked
- ½ cup of the grated Parmesan cheese
- Some salt to taste
- Some ground black pepper to taste
- 3 tablespoons of the extra virgin olive oil
- Some oil for spraying

Directions

- Preheat an oven at 450 degrees F
- Take a bowl add the breadcrumbs
- Then take a blender add the grated onions and blend them then pour them on the breadcrumbs including the juice so that the breadcrumbs are soaked
- Then add the rest of the ingredients into the bowl and stir them to combine all the ingredients
- Then add the salmon in the bowl mix them together and mix them by using your hands and make a thick paste like structure
- Then take n ice-cream scoop
- And extract the paste and make thick patties

and then set them aside
- Take a baking tray lined with parchment paper and drizzle some olive oil sprayed the oil all over the tray
- Then put the patties on the tray
- Let them bake for about 15 minutes
- After 15 minutes remove them and serve with the dipping sauce off your choice
- I have served with cauliflower puree and yogurt slaw
- Enjoy

Broccoli Rice

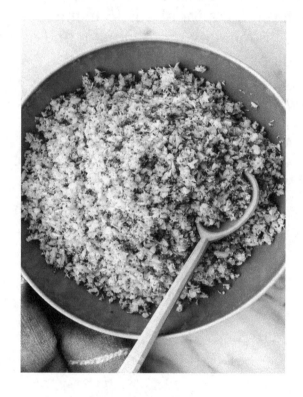

Prep Time: 10 minutes
Cook Time: 5 minutes
Servings: 4 people

Ingredients

- 8 ounces of the broccoli head
- 1 tablespoon of the extra virgin olive oil
- 3 scallions in diced form
- 1 minced garlic clove
- 2 tablespoons of the chopped cilantro
- Some salt to taste
- Some freshly ground black pepper to taste
- ¼ teaspoon of the cumin powder
- 1 tablespoon of lemon zest
- 1 tablespoon of lemon juice
- 1 cup of brown rice cooked

Directions

- Take a bowl and cut the broccoli florets in pieces then finely chopped them
- Drain them by using water. Take a food processor and process them in tiny rice shaped pieces
- Now take a nonstick skillet on the medium heat and brush them with some olive oil. Then add the riced broccoli, cilantro stems, garlic, scallions, some salt and ground black pepper. Let them cook for 5 minute then remove them in a plate and stir it with cumin powder, lemon juice and lemon zest.
- Then add the brown rice in them
- Stir them to combine and then serve them and enjoy

Roasted Brussels Sprouts

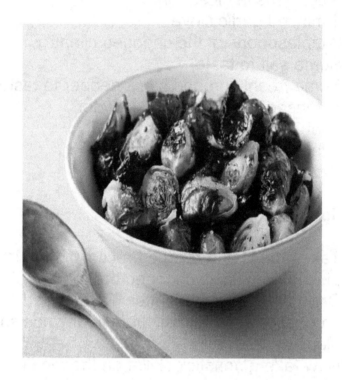

Prep Time: 10 minutes
Cook Time: 40 minutes
Serving: 6 people

Ingredients

- 2 pounds of the brussels sprouts
- 3 tablespoons of extra virgin olive oil
- Some kosher salt to taste
- Some ground black pepper to taste

Directions

- Preheat an oven at 450 degrees F
- Take a bowl and add the Brussels sprouts (cut it's ends and pull of its outer yellow leaves)
- The put them on the baking sheet sprayed with some olive oil and let them roast for 45 minutes until they are crispy and tendered from the inside
- Stir them occasionally for that the Brussels sprouts get brown evenly
- Then sprinkle them with some salt and black pepper to taste
- Then serve them immediately and enjoy

Anti-inflammatory Smoothie

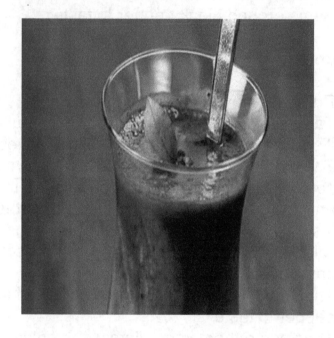

Prep Time: 5 minutes
Serving: 1 people

Ingredients

- 2 cups of loosely packed baby spinach
- 1 inch of ginger thinly sliced in minced form
- 1 bananas (frozen and cut into chunks)
- 1 mango peeled and diced
- ½ cup of beetroot juice
- ½ cup of skimmed milk
- 7 ice cubes

Directions

- Take a blender add all the ingredients together until well combined and smooth creamy smoothie is formed
- Serve them chilled and enjoy

Mango And Strawberries Smoothie

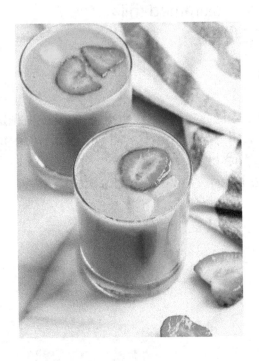

Prep Time: 5 minutes
Servings: 1 people

Ingredients

- 2 cups of sliced frozen strawberries
- 2 cups of mango peeled and in diced form
- 1 small carrot peeled and chopped
- 2 cups of the almond milk
- 1 teaspoon of Lemon juice
- ¼ cup of the orange juice

Directions

- Take a blender add all the ingredients together until well combined and smooth creamy smoothie is formed
- Serve them chilled and enjoy

Kale And Pineapple Smoothie

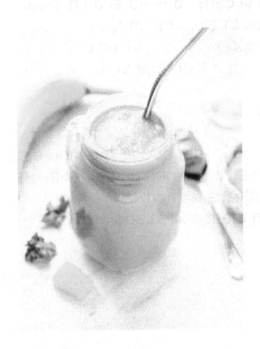

Prep Time: 5 minutes
Servings: 1 people

Ingredients

- 2 cups of washed and water drained kale leaves
- 2 cups of unsweetened vanilla milk
- 1 banana (frozen, peeled and cut into chunks)
- 3 tablespoons of Greek yogurt
- ¼ cup of the frozen pineapple chunks
- 2 tablespoons of the peanut butter
- 2 tablespoons of honey

Directions

- Take a blender add all the ingredients together until well combined and smooth creamy smoothie is formed
- Serve them chilled and enjoy

Chia And Pomegranate Smoothie

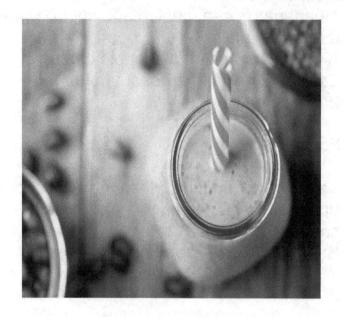

Prep Time: 5 minutes
Servings: 1 people

Ingredients

- 1 cup of any yogurt (I choose plain yogurt)
- 1 teaspoon of the Chia seeds
- ½ cup of pomegranate seeds
- 1 cup of the berries (frozen)
- 1 teaspoon of the stevia

Directions

- Take a blender add all the ingredients together until well combined and smooth creamy smoothie is formed
- Serve them chilled and enjoy

Oats And Berries Smoothie

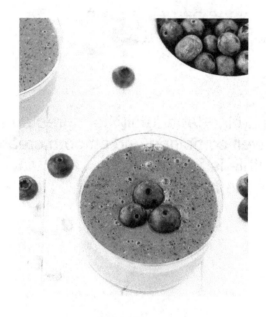

Prep Time: 5 minutes
Servings: 1 people

Ingredients

- 35 grams of the rolled oats
- 6 ounces of the Greek yogurt
- 120 grand of the blueberries (frozen)
- 2 cups of water
- 1 banana (frozen, peeled and cut into chunks)
- 5 ice cubes

Directions

- Take a blender add all the ingredients together until well combined and smooth creamy smoothie is formed
- Top then with frozen blueberries, serve them chilled and enjoy

Veggie Wraps with Cilantro Hummus

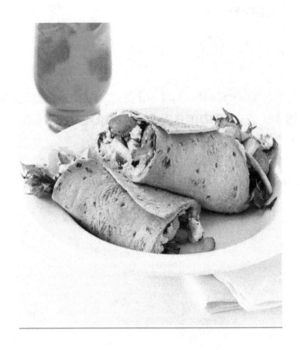

Prep Time: 10 minutes
Cook Time: 15 minutes
Servings: 2 people

Ingredients

- 1 cup of chopped cucumbers
- 1 cup of chopped cherry tomatoes
- 1 cup of boil chickpeas (skin removed or mixed with kosher salt and ground black pepper)
- 2 tablespoons of sesame paste
- 1 tablespoon of lemon juice
- 1 cup of cilantro leaves
- 1 tablespoon of white pepper powder
- 1 tablespoon of chopped garlic
- 2 tablespoons of chopped red onions
- 3 tablespoons of shredded Feta cheese
- 2 multi-grain wraps

Directions

Prepare Cilantro Hummus

- Take a food processor add minced garlic, chickpeas, lemon juice, olive oil, sesame seeds paste, some salt and white pepper
- Process them until it converts them int9 smooth form. Stop the processor and add cilantro and process them for 2 minutes until the cilantro is properly chopped
- Stop the processor and let the mixture cool
- To prepare the mediterranean wraps take a bowl add chopped cucumbers, cherry tomatoes, red onions and feta cheese. For the

dressing take a bowl add olive oil, vinegar, garlic and black pepper stir them until they get mixed

- Pour this dressing on the veggies toss them for 2 minutes to get them mixed
- Take a plate and spread each wrap with hummus. Top them with green veggies. Roll them and serve immediately
- Enjoy it

Lentil & Sweet Potatoes Patties

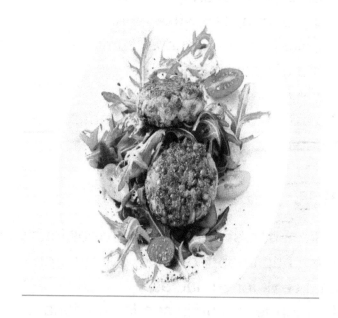

Prep Time: 15 minutes
Cook Time: 25 minutes
Servings: 2 people

Ingredients

- 2 tablespoons of olive oil
- 2 tablespoon of chopped garlic
- 1 cup of chopped white onions
- 1 tablespoon of turmeric, cumin and coriander
- 1 cup of baby spinach
- 1 cup of boil lentils
- 2 cups of mashed sweet potatoes
- 1 cup of corn flour

Directions

- Take a non-stick pan add olive oil let it warm up
- Then add chopped garlic, chopped onions and let it cook for 3 minutes
- Add turmeric, cumin seeds and coriander
- Mix it well
- Add baby spinach let it cook for 5 minutes after that remove from the flame
- Add these ingredients in a bowl and add lentils and mashed tomatoes
- Mix all the ingredients
- Make patties and coat them with corn flour
- Take a pan add olive oil and fry the patties from both sides
- Serve them with your favorite sauce and veggies

Chickpeas Patties

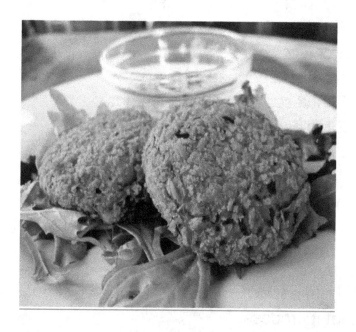

Prep Time: 15 minutes
Cook Time: 15 minutes
Servings: 2 people

Ingredients

- 1 ½ cup of boiled chickpeas
- Some kosher salt to taste
- 1 cup of chopped carrots
- 1 cup of chickpeas flour
- 1 cup of chopped onions
- 1 cup of chopped parsley
- 2 tablespoons of Psyllium husk
- 2 tablespoons of chopped garlic
- 2 tablespoons of paprika
- 1 tablespoon of cumin
- 3 tablespoons of tahini yum

Directions

- Take a food processor add the chickpeas and let it process
- After that remove it in a bowl and add all the ingredients in a bowl
- Mix all the ingredients with hands and then make patties
- Take a baking tray put parchment paper and spread the chickpeas flour coated patties and bake it for 10 minutes
- Serve it with your favourite sauce
- Enjoy it

Anti-inflammatory Appetizers

Anti-inflammatory Turmeric Bars

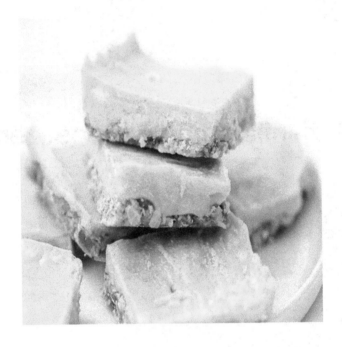

Prep Time: 10 minutes
Cook Time: 20 minutes
Servings: 6 people

Ingredients

- **For the crust**
- 1 cup of the shredded coconut
- 10 dates (pitted and let them soak in the water for about 10 minutes)
- 1 tablespoon of the coconut oil
- 1 teaspoon the cinnamon powder
- **For the filling**
- 1 ¼ cup of the coconut butter
- Half cup of the coconut oil
- 2 teaspoons of the turmeric powder
- 1 teaspoon of the cinnamon powder some extra for garnishing
- Some ground black pepper to taste
- 2 tablespoons of the maple syrup

Directions

- Preheat an oven and take a baking sheet lined with the parchment paper
- Take a food processor and add the pitted dates and shredded coconuts let them pulse until smooth mixture is formed
- Then add in coconut oil and cinnamon powder. Let them quickly blend
- Then spoon them in the pan and let them press by using the back of the spoon until they are flattened

- Transfer them in the fridge for about 3 hours
- Now make a filling by using the double broiler method
- Take a saucepan add the water in them turn on the flame and then put the small Stainless Steel bowl and add the coconut butter, let them melt
- Then stir in them the coconut oil stir then to combine well
- Then remove them from the heat and let them cool down
- Then stir in them the cinnamon powder, black pepper, turmeric powder, and maple syrup in them
- The pouring them on the crust and spread them evenly on the crust by using the spoon
- Place then in the refrigerator for overnight
- Then remove them from the fridge and set them aside
- Then cut them in the slices
- Then top them with the cinnamon powder
- Then store them in the refrigerator and then serve them and enjoy

Turmeric Gummies

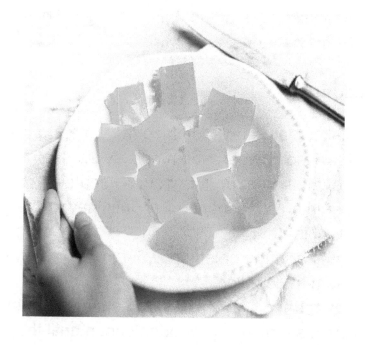

Prep Time: 4 hours and 10 minutes
Cook Time: 5 minutes
Servings: 4 people

Ingredients

- 3 ½ cup of the water
- 1 teaspoon of the ground turmeric
- 1 tablespoon of the maple syrup
- 8 tablespoons of the unflavored gelatin powder
- Some salt to taste

Directions

- Take a large pot, combine the water, ground turmeric powder, and maple syrup
- Let them heat up for about 5 minutes
- Let them stir continuously until they are fully combined
- Then add the gelatin powder in the pot and stir them to combine
- Then transfer them to the the heat, then let them stir by using wooden spoon until they are fully dissolved
- Then pour this mixture in the deep dish and cover them with a plastic wrap
- Then transfer them to the refrigerator, and let them chill for about 4 hours
- Once they are chilled then cut them into squares
- Then serve them and enjoy

Ginger Turmeric Bone Broth Protein Bites

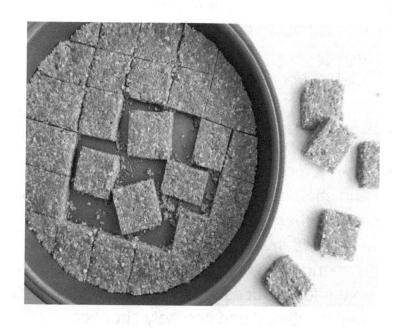

Prep Time: 10 minutes
Cook Time: 20 minutes
Servings: 20 people

Ingredients

- 1 cup of the raw cashews
- Half cup of the shredded coconuts
- 3 tablespoons of the unsweetened sunflower butter
- 2 tablespoons of the maple syrup
- 1 scoop of the organic turmeric bone broth protein
- 1 tablespoon of the ground ginger

Directions

- Take a food processor and add the cashews and shredded coconuts to the food processor and let them pulse until coarsely chopped
- Then add the sunflower butter, maple syrup, turmeric bone broth protein, and ground ginger to the food processor and let then pulse until well combined and coarsely chopped
- Then transfer this mixture to the pan and let them press by using your hands until they are firm and even layer
- Then transfer them to the refrigerator and let them set for about 20 minutes until they are firmed then cut them in the squares
- Then serve them and enjoy

Spicy Tuna Rolls

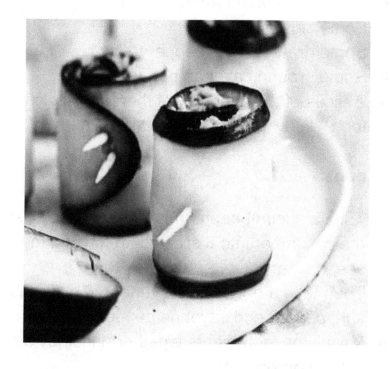

Prep Time: 10 minutes
Cook Time: 10 minutes
Servings: 6 people

Ingredients

- 1 medium sized cucumber
- 1 pound of the yellowish tuna
- 1 teaspoon of the red chilli sauce
- Some salt to taste
- Some ground black pepper to taste
- Some ground cayenne pepper to taste
- 2 slices of the avocado let them cut in diced form

Directions

- Take a cucumber and mandolin and thinly slice the cucumber into 6 slices by removing the seeds side
- Then take a bowl add the tuna, red chilli sauce, salt, pepper and cayenne pepper
- Mix all the ingredients together until they are fully incorporated
- Then take a slice of cucumber and spoon on them them the tuna mixture across it's slices
- Then carefully place each piece of the avocado on the tuna
- Then carefully roll up the cucumber by securing its end by using the toothpicks
- Then serve them and enjoy

Ginger Spiced Mixed Nuts

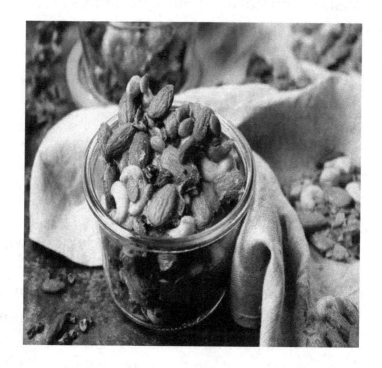

Prep Time: 5 minutes
Cook Time: 40 minutes
Servings: 8 people

Ingredients

- 2 golden eggs white
- 2 cups of the mixed nuts (raw almonds, cashew, pumpkin seeds, goji berries)
- 1 teaspoon of the finely grated ginger
- Some salt to taste
- Half teaspoon of the ground Vietnamese cinnamon
- Some coconut oil for spraying

Directions

- Preheat an oven at 259 degrees F
- Take take a bowl add eggs white let them whip until they are frothy
- Then add in them grated ginger, sea salt, and Vietnamese cinnamon, let them whipping until they are well combined
- Then add the nuts in the egg mixture and let them coat well
- Take a baking tray lined with parchment paper and spray them with some coconut oil
- Spread the nuts evenly over the baking tray
- Then transfer them to the oven and let them bake for about 40 minutes
- By rotating them half way through
- Then remove them from the oven and let them set aside

- Let them break into pieces and then serve them and enjoy

Spicy Kale Chips

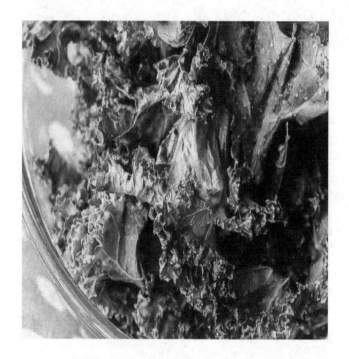

Prep Time: 8 minutes
Cook Time: 18 minutes
Servings: 4 people

Ingredients

- 1 large-sized bunch of the curly kale
- Some olive oil for spraying
- Some sea salt to taste
- Some cayenne pepper to taste
- Some ground black pepper to taste
- Some garlic powder to taste

Directions

- Preheat an oven at 450 degrees F
- Take a bowl and add the kale leaves let them rinsed with the clean water, then let them dry or pat then by using the paper towel to absorb the excess water
- Then year the kale leaves by using your hands into potato chips size
- Take a large sized baking sheet lined with parchment paper
- Put the kale torn leaves on the baking sheet then drizzle some olive oil and let them massage by using your hands and then sprinkle the remaining ingredients then toss them to coat well
- Transfer them to the baking oven and let them bake for about 20 minutes until they are crispy
- Then after that remove them from the oven and then serve them and enjoy

Ginger Date Bars

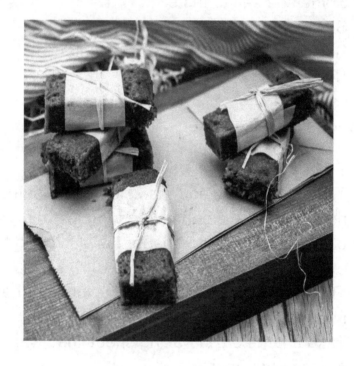

Prep Time: 20 minutes
Cook Time: 10 minutes
Servings: 8 people

Ingredients

- 2 cups of the the almonds
- 1 cup of the almond flour
- ¾ cup of the pitted medjool dates
- 5 tablespoons of the almond milk
- 1 teaspoon of the grated ginger

Directions

- Preheat an oven at 350 degrees F
- Take a high speed blender and add the almonds in them let them pulse until they are converted into powdery form then transfer them or the bowl and settlement aside
- Then in the same blender add the water soaked medjool dates along with the almond milk. Let them pulse until they are converted into paste form
- Then add the almond flour and grated ginger in the dates mixture
- Let them blend for about 4 minutes
- Let them cool down and then slice them in 8 bars
- Then transfer them to the refrigerator for about 1 hour then transfer them in the plate
- Serve them and enjoy

Vanilla Turmeric Orange Juice

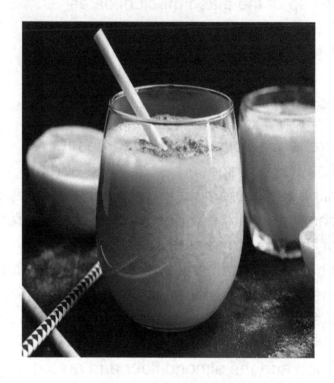

Prep Time: 5 minutes
Cook Time: 0 minute
Servings: 2 people

Ingredients

- 3 oranges peeled and let them cut in quarters size
- 1 cup of the unsweetened almond milk
- 1 teaspoon of the vanilla extract
- Half teaspoon of the ground cinnamon
- Half teaspoon of the ground turmeric powder
- Some pinch of black pepper to taste

Directions

- Take a high speed blender and add all the ingredients in them let them blend until they are well combined and smooth creamy smoothie type mixture is formed
- Pour them in the glass then serve them and enjoy

Ginger Gelatin Gummies

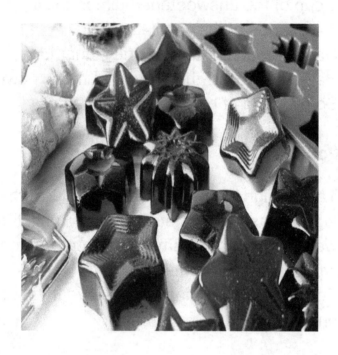

Prep Time: 10 minutes
Cook Time: 2 minutes
Servings: 28 people

Ingredients

- 1 cup of the filtered water
- 3 tablespoons of the hibiscus flowers cut
- 2 tablespoons of the honey
- 2 tablespoons of the ginger juice
- 2 tablespoons of the gelatin powder

Directions

- Take a small pot put them put the heat and add the water in it
- Then remove the water from the heat and add the hibiscus flowers
- Let them cover and infuse then for about 5 minutes
- Then drain the flowers with a strainer
- Then return the liquid to the pot, add the ginger and honey. Let them mix
- Then sprinke the gelatin powder over the liquid and let them soften and dissolve
- Then give them a whisk so that n9 clumps remain behind
- Pour this mixture in the silicone mold
- Let them transfer to the fridge for about 2 hours
- Then remove them and serve

Baked Veggies Turmeric Nuggets

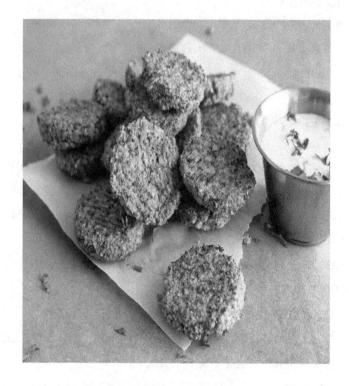

Prep Time: 25 minutes
Cook Time: 10 minutes
Servings: 24 people

Ingredients

- 2 cups of the cauliflower florets
- 2 cups of the broccoli florets
- 1 cup of the carrot coarsely chopped
- 1 teaspoon of the minced garlic
- Half teaspoon of the ground turmeric powder
- Some salt to taste
- Some ground black pepper to taste
- Half cup of the almond meal
- 1 large sized golden egg

Directions

- Preheat an oven at 450 degrees F
- Take a baking tray lined with parchment paper
- Take a food processor and add all the ingredients except the egg and let them pulse until they are coarsely chopped or ground
- Then after that crack the egg in them and again pulse them for 2 minutes
- Transfer this mixture to the bowl and then make patties by using your wet hands
- Then put these patties on the parchment lined baking tray
- Let them bake for about 25 minutes until they turned into golden brown and crispy
- Then serve them with the paleo ranch dressing
- Enjoy

Creamy Pineapple Ginger Slaw

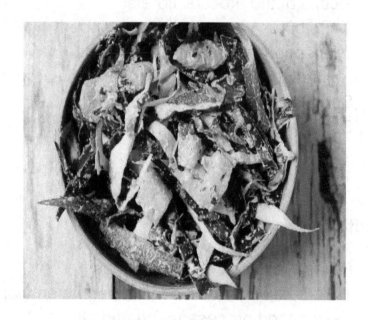

Prep Time: 40 minutes
Cook Time: 0 minute
Servings: 12 people

Ingredients

Creamy Ginger Sauce

- 1 cup of the soaked cashew
- Half cup of the water
- 2 tablespoons of the lemon juice
- 2 teaspoons of the fresh ginger
- Half teaspoon of the red pepper flakes
- Some salt to taste
- Some ground black pepper to taste

Pineapple Slaw

- Half head of the red cauliflower thinly sliced
- Half head of the green cabbage thinly sliced
- 2 red peppers thinly sliced
- 3 cups of the pineapple cut them in small chunks
- 1 cup of the roughly chopped cilantro leaves

Directions

- Take a bowl add water and cashews in them. Let them soak for overnight
- Take a food processor and add all the sauce ingredients and the soaked cashews
- Let them pulse until they converted into smooth sauce mixture

- Take a bowl add the red cabbage, green cabbage, red peppers and pineapple chunks
- Then drizzle the sauce over them
- Stir them to combine and coat well with the rest of the ingredients
- Then add the cilantro leaves and then stir them to incorporate
- Then serve them and enjoy

Turmeric Coconut Flour Muffins

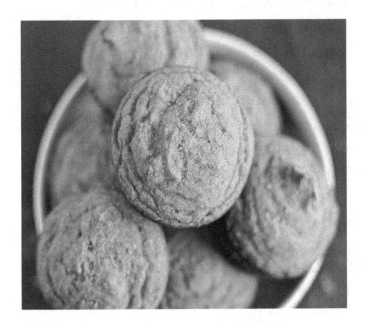

Prep Time: 25 minutes
Cook Time: 5 minutes
Servings: 8 people

Ingredients

- 6 large golden eggs
- Half cup of the unsweetened coconut milk
- 3 tablespoons of the maple syrup
- 1 teaspoon of the vanilla extract
- ¾ cup of the coconut flour
- 2 tablespoons of the coconut flour
- Half teaspoon of the baking soda
- 2 teaspoons of the turmeric powder
- Half teaspoon of the ginger powder
- Some salt and black pepper to taste

Directions

- Preheat an oven at 450 degree F
- Take a muffin tin and line them with the parchment paper
- Then take a bowl, crack golden eggs, add milk, vanilla extract, and maple syrup. Stir them to combine well until the start to bubble
- Take another bowl add the coconut flour, vanilla extract, baking soda, turmeric powder, ginger powder, salt and pepper
- Start stirring the dry ingredients with the wet ingredients and make a thick batter
- Then transfer this batter to the muffin tins evenly

- Transfer them to the baking oven and let them bake for about 25 minutes until they are turned into golden brown
- Then remove the muffins from the oven and then serve them and enjoy

Golden Turmeric Energy Bites

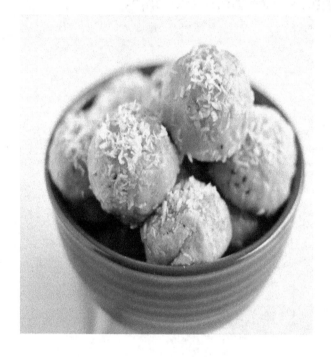

Prep Time: 5 hours
Cook Time: 20 minutes
Servings: 18 people

Ingredients

- 1 cup of the almond butter
- ¾ cup of the unsweetened coconut flakes
- 6 tablespoons of the protein powder
- 1 teaspoon of the coconut oil
- Half teaspoon of the maple syrup
- 2 teaspoons of the turmeric powder

Directions

- Take a blender add the nuts butter, coconut flakes, almond butter, coconut oil, maple syrup, protein powder and turmeric powder
- Blend the ingredients until they are well combined together
- Let the dough transfer to the refrigerator to make it harden
- Then remove the dough from the refrigerator and make balls
- Then put them on the plate lined with parchment paper
- Transfer them to the refrigerator for about 3 hours
- Then remove the balls from the refrigerator and sprinkle on them coconut flakes
- Then serve them and enjoy

Ginger Fried Cabbage And Carrots

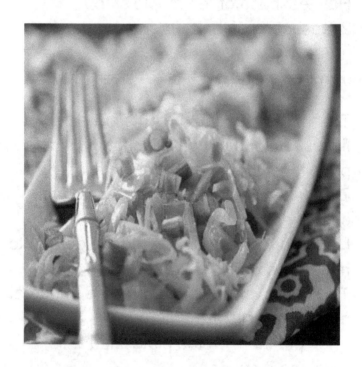

Prep Time: 5 minutes
Cook Time: 8 minutes
Servings: 15 people

Ingredients

- 2 tablespoons of the extra virgin olive oil
- 1 tablespoon of the minced ginger
- 2 minced garlic cloves
- 4 cups of the shredded green cabbage
- 2 carrots julienned or grated
- 1 tablespoon of the apple cider vinegar
- 1 tablespoon of the coconut aminos
- ¼ cup of the green onions, chopped

Directions

- Take a nonstick pan add the oil then add the garlic and ginger let them saute for 3 minutes until they are tendered or turned into golden brown and their fragrance comes out
- Then add the cabbage and carrot let them cook for about 8 mimutes
- After 8 minutes remove the cabbage from the stove and then stir in them coconut aminos, vinegar and green onions
- Stir them to combine and then serve them and enjoy

Turmeric Ginger Smoothie With Coconut Oil

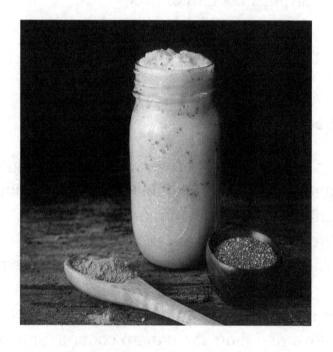

Prep Time: 5 minutes
Cook Time: 0 minute
Servings: 1 people

Ingredients

- 2 cups of the unsweetened almond milk
- 1 teaspoon of the turmeric powder
- 1 teaspoon of the melted coconut oil
- 2 tablespoons of the pure honey
- 1 teaspoon of the ginger peeled and finely chopped
- 1 teaspoon of the chia seeds
- 6 ice cubes

Directions

- Take a high speed blender and add all the ingredients except the chia seeds and let them blend until well combined
- Then pour them in the glass and stir in them the chia seeds let them set aside for about 5 minutes to bloom the chia seeds
- Then serve them and enjoy

Grain Free Banana Ginger Bars

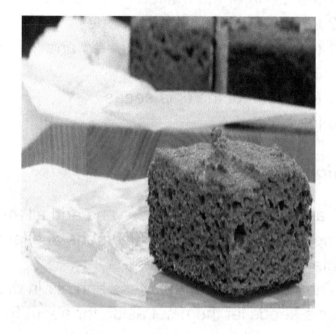

Prep Time: 10 minutes
Cook Time: 40 minutes
Servings: 4 people

Ingredients

- 2 large sized ripe bananas
- 1 cup of the coconut flour
- 3 tablespoons of the coconut flour
- 6 golden eggs
- 2 tablespoons of the freshly grated ginger
- 2 teaspoons of the ground cinnamon powder
- 2 teaspoons of the ground cardamom
- 1 teaspoon of the baking powder
- 2 teaspoons of the apple cider vinegar

Directions

- Preheat an oven at 350 degrees F
- Take a glass baking dish lined with the parchment paper
- Then take a food processor and add all the ingredients except baking soda and vinegar. Let them combine until they are pulsed together
- After that add the baking soda and vinegar
- Then pour them on the glass baking dish
- Transfer them to the baking oven and let them bake for about 40 minutes
- Then remove them and cut them in slices and enjoy

Thank you!

We have given you the best recipes to add to your diet to relive your chronic disease and inflammation

CPSIA information can be obtained
at www.ICGtesting.com
Printed in the USA
BVHW062328150621
609638BV00012B/1021